Nathan's Story

~Insights from the Life of Our Miracle Child~

By Cheryl Smith Benefield

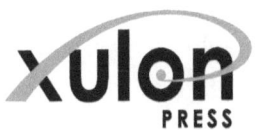

DEDICATION

—∿—

This book is dedicated to
Nathan Lee Benefield
the "Miracle Child" God gave us,
and whose life story has blessed so many.

For God said:
Before I formed you in the womb, I knew you,
before you were born, I set you apart...
(Jeremiah 1:5)

ACKNOWLEDGEMENTS

—᠕᠕—

To my parents, Rev. Rudolph and Mrs. Edna L. Smith, "Papa and Granny": I could not have made it through these past 14 years without your love, support, and encouragement as you assisted with the care of Nathan. I am eternally grateful to you, Granny. Four months after Nathan was born, you retired as a registered nurse so you could become one of his primary care givers. Nathan deeply loves you and Papa, and enjoys spending time with you.

To my two older children, Edwin and Stefani: You have always been supportive of Nathan and loved him unconditionally. Since your dad's death you have filled in the gap and assisted me with Nathan's care, discipline, and developmental strategies. Even in the midst of your pain and loss, you committed to focusing on meeting the needs of your little brother. You emphatically stated that your commitment is not out of duty but love because he is your brother. I am so proud of how you have assumed responsibilities for Nathan, and I love you both very much.

To my Auntie Willie Maude and my Big Mama: After Nathan came home from the hospital and had so many therapy and doctor appointments, you joined mom in making those many trips around I-285 to the Scottish Rite Medical Facility (now Children's Healthcare of Atlanta) whenever Earnest and I could not take him. Auntie, you have simply amazed me with your resolve to be an active care giver for Nathan when he was younger. I have watched God strengthen your faith and enhance your care-giving skills. Big Mama, your unconditional love for all of us also embraced Nathan with whom you developed a special bond.

To Peaches, "Godmama": You asked for the honor to become his godmother and were determined to expose him to some of life's best adventures. Your love for Nathan has been demonstrated by your actions, the trips to the state parks, the vacations to Hilton Head, and much more.

To my brother Michael and his wife, Felecia, my nephew Allan and niece Allyson: Your love and encouragement have sustained us many a day.

To my extended support system and prayer warriors – Auntie Irma, Sybil, Vivian, Bernadine, Cynthia and many others, especially the family of Community Church of God: Your love, encouragement, and prayers made it possible for us to move forward, survive this journey, and hold fast to our faith.

To all Nate's teachers – Marti Kennedy, Cathy Duncan, Edna Wilson, C. A. Edwards, Cheryl Eaton, Ellen Dollar, Elisha Gray, and all the paraprofessionals, therapists, and medical doctors, especially Leonard Sacks, Valerie Wright-Manley, Loreen Doyle-Little, Glenda Morris-Robinson, LeRoy Graham, and Olga Sherrod, who have worked with Nathan these past 14 years: Your contributions to his life are more significant than you will ever know.

To my lifelong friends, Johnnie R. Miller and Susan Coronis: I am grateful to you for agreeing to edit this book. I value our friendship and your professionalism.

To everyone who contributed to the section, *"Lessons Learned from Nathan & Special Moments"*: Thank you for your responses and insights.

Finally to my accountability "sistahs", Maggie and Shon: We share a special sisterhood bond and you have held me accountable for completing this book. You helped me maintain my focus and determination to complete this book by December 2008. I love you and am grateful for our sisterhood, and because of you, the mission is accomplished.

During these past 14 years of Nathan's life, so many people have spoken encouraging words, demonstrated their love to us and prayed with and for us. Your love and prayers have strengthened our family more than you will ever know.

May God continue to bless everyone who has been involved in Nathan's life and whose lives Nathan has touched.

TABLE OF CONTENTS

—◦◦◦—

FOREWORD

—〰—

This book is the story of a pilgrimage of faith. It is an account of an unshaken faith of a mother in the promises and power of God that eventuated into miracles that we witness even now.

Nathan's birth was a miracle itself, the result of my daughter's faith to trust God in the face of preliminary medical reports that the odds were against her unborn child surviving a multiplicity of complications. In the face of these dire medical diagnoses, Cheryl remained steadfast in her trust in God's promises.

During those difficult days of Nathan's postnatal and neonatal care, Cheryl's faith and hope sustained us to trust God also and to believe that God, in His infinite wisdom, had chosen to entrust this special child in our care.

As a family we have been blessed to see his growth and development. Though his expressive language is limited, Nathan can communicate in other ways. We continue to marvel at his amazing memory. Though mentally challenged, he can obey simple instructions. Like all children, Nathan desires and responds to love and affection. Hugs and kisses are the order of the day.

The lessons we have learned from Nathan are to live life with thanksgiving to God, with gratitude for His blessings, and with humility in serving others. May this book be a blessing to all who read it, especially those who must care for special needs children.

Rev. Dr. Rudolph Smith (Papa)

PROLOGUE

—ᴠᴠ—

*"For I know the plans I have for you," declares
the Lord, "plans to prosper you and not to harm
you, plans to give you hope and a future. Then you
will call upon me and come and pray to me, and
I will listen to you. You will seek me and find me
when you seek me with all your heart."*
(Jeremiah 29:11-13)

This book has been a work in progress since the unexpected death of my husband Earnest in August 2005. Our youngest child Nathan, with his special needs, has transformed our life. He and his dad shared a special bond. For several years prior to Earnest's death, I had been thinking about telling *Nathan's Story*: how God had given him to us, the miracles God performed in his life, and how Nathan has transformed so many lives. However, I failed to make it a priority until after my husband died. Then my priorities changed, and in December 2005 I sensed a need to begin recording and documenting *Nathan's Story*.

Since his birth, we have called Nathan our *"miracle baby"* because God performed the first miracle of his life while he was in my womb. Two weeks after the doctors saw at least seven holes in his heart on a sonogram, God closed them. After he was born, this miracle was manifested, and the doctors were baffled. Throughout the years, God has performed other miracles in Nathan's life, which have strengthened our faith, knitted our family closer together, and encouraged others.

So this book is written to provide encouragement and inspiration for those families who have been blessed with the opportunity to nurture and raise children who have special needs. When God places a special needs child within our families, we need to recognize we have been blessed with a gift, for we have been counted worthy to care for and to raise that child.

As parents, our role is to love and nurture these children and to provide them with the best possible care. I know the journey has many challenges, but God is able to strengthen us and provide the necessary resources along the way.

My family and I have been blessed to meet many people who have assisted us with Nathan's care and developmental needs. Without Nathan, we would have missed opportunities to develop relationships and discover resources that were available to him and other special needs children. Truly, Nathan is our gift from God. Through him, God has demonstrated His power of healing, the power of prayer, and the power of genuine love.

May all who read this book be encouraged and blessed. May you discover the opportunities you have to be a blessing to others and profoundly understand that all children are gifts from God. Even though the journey may become tedious, if we trust God, He will provide for our every need, strengthen us for our daily journey and empower us to do His will.

For we know "*nothing is impossible with God*" (Luke1:37), and we give Him all praise and glory for what He has done in Nathan's life.

Be blessed!

MEDICAL MIRACLES & SIGNIFICANT EVENTS

—ɷ—

"But God chose the foolish things of the world to shame the wise; God chose the weak things of the world to shame the strong. He chose the lowly things of this world and the despised things – and the things that are not – to nullify the things that are, so that no one may boast before Him."
(I Corinthians 1:27-29)

In the year of our Lord, 1994, God decided to send one of His special angels to earth to be a blessing to all he would meet. The Lord knew that this little angel would change the lives of many people and lead them to a greater knowledge of the power of God. He also knew that this little angel would cause people to recognize the love of God.

Prior to his arrival, we had been told that our little angel would have special needs, and I was given the option to have an abortion. However, because I trusted God, I chose to give life to God's special angel. I told the doctors that we would love the child that God had chosen to give us, no matter what the sonogram predicted. I also refused the doctors' request for amniocentesis to confirm their suspicions. They told me he would be born with Down syndrome, and predicted that he also would be born with at least seven holes in his heart, which would require multiple surgeries to correct. Nevertheless, after receiving such dismal news, I was resolute in my determination to give birth to the angel God had sent us.

When I left the doctor's office that day in June, I cried all the way back to my school. I told my assistant principal I had not received good news from the doctor, and I asked to go home early so that I could regain my composure. Our high school graduation ceremony was that evening and since I was the SGA sponsor, I needed to be there to support my students.

After I went home and shared the news with my husband, we decided not to tell our children until the baby was born. I called my parents to relay the news. Then I decided to share the report with only a few close family members and friends who were asked to pray with us.

Two weeks later I went to work at our church's state youth camp because I wanted to maintain my regular summer activities as much as possible. After I came home from camp, I became ill during the night. I had no idea what was happening to me so I began to pray. As I prayed, the Lord spoke to me in a still, small voice and revealed that He was healing the baby in my womb. I became excited and thought that Nathan would be a healthy baby.

So on August 28, 1994, God dispatched his special angel to earth, making his arrival nine weeks premature according to man's timetable. But on God's schedule, he was right on time. Weighing in at three pounds and 13.8 ounces, our little angel arrived and was named Nathan Lee Benefield. His cousin Allan chose the name Nathan, which means "Gift of God", and I chose to give him his dad's middle name, Lee. We affectionally called him "Nate". God sent this little angel to the household of Earnest Lee and Cheryl Louise Smith Benefield, because He entrusted us to provide all the tender loving care our special baby would need.

After Nathan was born, I discovered the Lord had healed his heart early that Sunday morning in June while he was still in my womb. After the pediatric cardiologist examined him, he came into my room and told my dad and me that he found no defects in Nathan's heart. He further stated that he was not sure why there were concerns about his heart. I explained to him that the earlier sonogram had shown at least seven holes in his heart, and he responded that Nathan's heart looked like a normal baby's heart. Dad and I began to praise the Lord and the cardiologist said that we "knew the right man".

Although we were elated with the good news about Nathan's heart, all the reports were not as good. Samples of his blood were sent to Emory University for a chromosome evaluation. Later the test results confirmed that Nathan had Down syndrome, which is officially called Trisonomy 21. Since it is not uncommon for babies with Down syndrome to have heart defects, we knew God had truly performed a miracle in Nathan's life when He healed his heart in my womb.

Nathan was also born with a blocked bowel and had to have corrective surgery (duodenum atresia) when he was three days old. Knowing that he might need a blood transfusion, I went to the Red Cross to give my own blood the day before the surgery. I could make this donation only because Nathan was born through natural child birth, without any drugs. Of my three pregnancies, his was the first in which I experienced natural child birth. I was determined that if he needed a blood transfusion, it would be with my blood.

Because he was a preemie, Nathan was placed in the Neonatal Intensive Care Unit at Piedmont Hospital in Atlanta, GA. His surgery went well, but we were told that he would have to stay in NICU for nine weeks or until he reached five pounds. But praise God, Nathan only stayed in NICU for 28 days. Every day, other family members and I visited him. The staff told me because they had observed the love and care we gave Nathan, they would let him come home when he reached four and a half pounds. They felt assured that he would be well cared for. One requirement for his release from the hospital was for Nathan to have a hearing test. Although the test was not conclusive, the result was not favorable.

Nathan came home on a fall morning in September after my husband and I, his Granny and

Auntie Willie Maude went through CPR training. It was a requirement because he was coming home on an Apnea monitor, and the possibility existed that he could stop breathing during the night. Surprisingly, Auntie learned the CPR technique better than I did. This woman, who was once known as the cry baby in our family and could not tolerate pain, stepped up to the plate and gave yeomen service to baby Nate; she became one of his active caregivers.

Although I was a special education teacher for 18 years, all of my work had been at the high school level; therefore, I had limited knowledge about services available for infants and toddlers. After Nathan was born, one of the pediatric nurses told me about the Marcus Center that serves Down syndrome children; she referred me to the hospital social worker who informed me about the Babies Can't Wait Program, an early intervention program for children with special needs. I also learned about the Katie Beckett Deeming Waiver which allows families to apply for Medicaid for children with special needs.

When he was two months old, Nathan had his first evaluation at the Marcus Center. He received services from the Babies Can't Wait program until he was three; then they transitioned him to a special pre-k program in the public schools. Through this early intervention program, we were assigned a case worker who made home visits and provided information about available resources and services. Nathan also received home visits from a representative of Georgia Pines which provides services for infants and children who are hearing impaired.

We were blessed to have a case worker who assisted me with the Katie Beckett Deeming Waiver application, arranged Nathan's evaluation at the Marcus Center and his initial placement at the REACH Center, and initiated his physical therapy sessions at Scottish Rite Children's Hospital. Once Nate was approved for the Katie Beckett Deeming Waiver, he obtained Medicaid benefits. All of these services were essential. Because of his medical conditions, Nate required several medications, some specialized equipment, and extensive therapies during his early years.

At 10 weeks old Nathan began receiving physical therapy because he had such low muscle tone, also known as hypotonia. It was painful for me to know my baby could not raise his head or turn over, but we were determined to give Nate all the necessary therapies to help him develop. As he progressed with his physical therapy, his speech limitations became more prominent. At six months, after intensive testing, Nathan was diagnosed with a sensorineural hearing loss in the inner ear, leaving little hope that he would ever talk. His diagnosis of "profoundly deaf" was confirmed shortly thereafter. One evening at church, during a performance of a children's choir from South Africa, we noticed that when the drums were played loudly, Nathan did not respond to any of the sounds.

As a result of his severe hearing loss, speech therapy was added to his treatment plan. Two months later, occupational therapy was added to address his fine and visual motor skills deficiencies. The goal was to ensure Nate had every therapy available to treat his developmental delays.

Among the doctors we needed to see was a pediatric ENT doctor. During a follow-up visit, when he was two, Dr. Thomson noted that Nathan's ear canals had opened up, which is very unusual for Down syndrome babies. But praise God, after his ear canals opened up, Nathan demonstrated more sensitivity to sounds. When his name was called, he eventually would say "huh". His receptive language improved, although his expressive language was limited. Nathan began to pay attention to his surroundings more and eventually began to respond to sounds. Later, he communicated with us by pointing, gesturing and taking us to whatever he wanted.

Without a doubt, we knew God had performed another miracle in Nathan's life. Shortly after receiving the news about his ear canals, we went on vacation to Hilton Head Island. While there, Stefani was playing her saxophone and hit a high note. Nathan screamed! He had never responded to sound like that before.

Early on we made a decision to try to teach Nathan some specific signs to help him with his communication. He easily mastered "hi" and "bye", and learned to sign "eat", "drink" and "more". Later, the "potty" sign was added to his vocabulary. Nate received his first hearing aids when he was two, but they made little difference in his responses. When he was eight, new hearing aids were made which amplified sounds more for him.

"Miracle Baby" is what our family affectionally began to call Nathan. First, the Lord healed his heart in my womb and brought him through duodenum atresia surgery at three days old. Then at three months old, God proved that Nathan did not need a liver biopsy.

When Nate's eyes became slightly jaundiced, the doctor expressed concern about his liver function and scheduled a liver biopsy. On the day of the biopsy, they could not find a vein to insert the I.V. Since Nathan was so small, his veins often rolled and collapsed, and it was sometimes difficult to draw blood from him or insert an I.V. However, when the phlebotomist drew his blood earlier that day, she collected an extra vial. I remember her saying that since his blood was flowing so well, she would fill an extra one. So, the doctors were able to take that vial and conduct the necessary tests to determine his liver function, and the results indicated no problems with his liver function. I know God was in control that day when the extra tube of blood was drawn.

Shortly thereafter, Nathan developed gastro esophageal reflux, which led to several bouts of pneumonia and hospitalizations. After repeated hospitalizations, we were advised that he needed to have surgery to insert a g-tube in his stomach for feeding or he could aspirate and die. We were told he would need the g-tube for feedings indefinitely until his oral motor skills improved. Nathan's low muscle tone contributed to his reflux because it affected his ability to suck and swallow appropriately. His inability to properly suck and swallow was identified as oral motor dysfunction.

So at the time, which I deemed was God's timing, his father and I consented to the surgery in April 1996. At the age of 16 months, God brought him through fundiplication and hernia surgery. As a result of this surgery, Nathan had a g-tube inserted into his stomach so he could take-in liquids to control his reflux and alleviate the fear of his aspirating. While he was recovering in the ICU unit, we saw further evidence of God's timing. His Papa prayed for a Finnish little girl who was also in the ICU, and whom the doctors did not give much hope of surviving. But God raised her up.

In the midst of all these events, God placed Christian care givers and doctors and therapists in Nathan's life. Specifically, Dr. LeRoy Graham, his pulmonologist, Dr. Olga Sherrod, his gastroenterologist and Dr. Theodore Atkinson, his developmental pediatrician always encouraged us to trust God. Amazingly, we met Dr. Graham during Nate's first visit to Scottish Rite's emergency room where he diagnosed him with pneumonia. Even though it was a painful way to meet Dr. Graham, we know it was all a part of God's plan. In his compassion, Dr. Graham later referred us to Dr. Atkinson who specialized in working with developmentally delayed children. And when the pneumonia kept reoccurring, we were referred to Dr. Sherrod for the treatment of Nathan's reflux. For several years, these specialists provided exceptional care for Nathan.

EDUCATIONAL OPPORTUNITIES & LIFE TRANSITIONS

—⁂—

"And we know that in all things God works for the good of those who love him, who have been called according to His purpose." (**Romans 8:28**)

Through the early intervention program, Nathan received his initial day care services at the REACH Center until he turned three. There he also received physical therapy, occupational therapy and speech therapy, and he was introduced to sign language. During his time at REACH, he had his first hearing evaluation at the Atlanta Area School for the Deaf, which continued on a regular basis until he was ten.

When Nathan turned three, he was released from the Babies Can't Wait Program, left the REACH Center and was placed in a half-day program at L. P. Miles Elementary School. His teacher, Ms. Cathy

Duncan, provided outstanding and loving care the two years he was there. During that time Nathan could not walk, received g-tube feedings, and began exhibiting self stimulating behavior – he would pull at his ears. Consequently, Nathan sometimes wore arm restraints to keep him from pulling at his ears. When he left Ms. Duncan's class, Nate spent the rest of the afternoon at MARDS (Metropolitan Atlanta Respite & Developmental Services, Inc.), a center that catered to special needs children.

After Nathan left the REACH Center, one of the challenges we faced was finding a quality program on the southside of Atlanta for special needs children. Not many day care centers were willing to work with this population of children. MARDS was the only place available. They offered summer programs, day care and weekend respite services. Nathan attended the MARDS summer program until 2005.

In his transition from pre-k to kindergarten, Nathan lost a year of progressing toward his IEP (Individualized Education Plan) goals when he was placed in an OI (Orthopedically Impaired) program with a teacher who really did not want to work with him. During most of the school day, Nathan sat in his wheelchair and received limited instruction until the therapists came to work with him.

The next year I investigated more suitable programs for him and had him placed at Cleveland Avenue Elementary School in Ms. Edna Wilson's class. That summer Nathan had Ms. Wilson as his ESY (Extended School Year) teacher. The following school year, under Ms. Wilson's guidance, Nathan graduated from the wheelchair to the walker and began walking independently. He was now six and a half years old. He also began participating in adaptive PE activities (including bowling), Special Olympics, and was integrated into some other school-wide activities.

Nathan really enjoyed participating in Special Olympics. The year after he started walking independently, he was ahead in his race until the crowd started clapping to cheer him on. Hearing the applause and the cheers, Nathan stopped walking and started clapping for himself. His response to the crowd cost him the lead. As he stopped to clap for himself the other participants passed him. Clapping is positive reinforcement for Nathan. When he does something right and we clap for him, he also claps for himself.

Once Nathan started walking, he liked to turn the lights off and on, open and close doors, and go out the door. In Ms. Wilson's class, he watched the staff to see what they were doing before attempting to do the things he should not. Sometimes, Nathan would refuse to do some of the tasks he needed to do. However, Ms. Wilson knew how to manage him by providing a structured environment, and Nathan soon learned who was in charge. We all learned that we needed to be consistent and firm with Nathan to make him cooperate.

After Nathan started walking, I decided to potty train him. By the time he was nine, he was wearing regular underwear and was significantly accident free. Once he learned the "potty" sign, sometimes Nathan would continually give the sign to make us move, even when he did not need to go. He learned quickly which family member or school personnel he could manipulate with the "potty" sign.

By the summer of 2000, Nathan had graduated from his g-tube feedings and was eating and drinking normally. While he had the G-tube button, it had to be replaced on an average of every two to three months, and periodically Nathan would undergo swallow studies to see if he were still aspirating or prone to aspirate. After four years of tube feedings, I decided not to replace the g-tube button when it came out the last time. This decision was made because the April 2000 swallow study, which was conducted prior to the g-tube button coming out, showed little possibility of aspiration. His muscle tone had improved a great deal, and I was trusting God that Nathan was healed and he would be all right. Now eight years later, Nathan eats and drinks whatever he wants without any problems.

While Nate was at Cleveland Avenue, he annually received his class "Most Improved Student Award". In the spring of 2005, Nathan participated in the fifth grade promotion exercise, walked across the stage and received his certificate. Some people were amazed that he sat in the regular chair for the duration of the ceremony. However, we were not because Nathan sits in church every Sunday.

Nathan's transition to middle school came one week after his father's unexpected death in August 2005. Many wondered if he understood that his father was gone because he had been the one who, in the mornings, had prepared Nathan's breakfast, dressed him for school, put him on the school bus, and took him off in the afternoon. After school, his father frequently took Nathan for afternoon rides in his truck. We really did not know if Nathan understood his father was gone, even though we had taken him to the funeral and he was the first one to throw his flower onto the casket at the grave.

Nathan and his dad developed a special bond after Earnest retired on disability in 1997. Earnest then assumed some of the responsibilities for taking Nate to Scottish Rite Medical Center for his PT and OT appointments. He often remarked how Nate enjoyed riding in the truck and looking out the window. He also said Nate would babble most of the way home from his appointments. For several years, they both enjoyed this special time together.

So, did Nathan know something was different and a change had occurred? Although he could not talk, Nathan was very observant. He was also a child who responded well to routine, and he had become accustomed to his dad being at home with him.

We soon learned that he did understand. He started middle school on Monday, two days after the funeral. That morning, I got him ready for school, put him on the bus, and took him off in the afternoon. The next day, his Auntie Sybil met the bus and walked him up the driveway to the house. When they got to the door, Nathan refused to come in; he looked at his daddy's truck parked in the driveway and began crying.

A week later, on a Saturday morning after I had fixed his breakfast and said grace, Nathan looked at me and said, "Bye-bye Dada." He had not said "dada" in some years. But he knew the big black truck that he loved to ride in had not moved in two weeks and that his daddy had not been home to do things with him and for him. Since his routine had changed, Nathan had figured out something was different. It seemed as if God had allowed him to express himself very clearly so we would know that he understood his daddy would not be coming back.

Nathan's transition to middle school was also impacted by the transition at home. Fortunately, his big sister Stefani had just graduated from college and was able to step in and assume the responsibilities of getting Nathan ready for school. His big brother Edwin also played a major role in helping with Nathan's care. He took Nate for rides in the truck and to various play activities. He and Stefani also became Nate's barber. I was concerned that since I was still working that I might be imposing on them to help me with Nathan. However, they assured me that caring for Nate was not an imposition because he was their little brother and they loved him. Together, the three of us worked as a team to make sure Nathan had a smooth transition from home to school.

As a family, we were very pleased that for the first time, Nathan would be attending his neighborhood school. It was the same school Edwin and Stefani had attended – Ralph Bunche Middle School. His teacher, Ms. Ellen Dollar, whom I had observed and selected earlier in the spring, and her paraprofessionals partnered with us to help Nate make this transition. She worked diligently with him for three years to help him achieve his IEP goals. Under her tutelage, he improved his sorting skills and recognition of colors. Nathan loved music, working on the computer and using the communication board, but he did not like activities in which he had to manipulate pencils or crayons. Ms. Dollar also designated Nate as her helper and assigned him specific tasks to do. While at Bunche Middle School, Nathan enjoyed Adaptive PE, (including swimming and bowling) and participating in the Special Olympics. During his last year at Bunche, he finally won first place in his race in the Special Olympics because he did not stop walking until he crossed the finish line. We knew then that Nathan was maturing and becoming focused.

In August 2008, Nathan entered high school. Again I investigated the two sites offering his special program and chose Maynard Jackson H.S. and Mrs. Elisha Gray as his teacher. Although I was a bit apprehensive about this transition to high school, my apprehension was allayed during the first three months of school because Nathan adapted to the high school environment. He enjoys working on the computer, Adaptive P.E. and the Community Based Learning experiences. Nathan still challenges the staff there by opening and closing doors, trying to go places he should not, and swiping food. But his teacher reports she, like his previous teachers, has found him to be very loving, yet energetic.

OVERCOMING CHALLENGES & AMAZING PROGRESS

—ɯ—

*"Now to Him who is able to do immeasurably
more than all we ask or imagine, according to His
power that is at work within us, to Him be glory
in the church and in Christ Jesus throughout all
generations, forever and ever! Amen."*
(Ephesians 3:20-21)

Truly, Nathan is a "miracle child" who was born
with Down syndrome, diagnosed initially as
profoundly deaf, and given little expectation to ever
walk or talk because he was severely hypotonic and
had a sensorineural hearing loss. Subsequently, he
was labeled as developmentally delayed. However,
after extensive and intensive physical therapy and
much prayer, Nathan sat up alone when he was two,
pulled himself up at four, and started walking independently when he was six and a half years old.

Once Nathan became mobile, he was an active ball of energy, as if he were making up for lost time. He would go from room to room opening doors, especially the bathroom where he would flush the toilet and turn the water on. He would also open kitchen cabinets and take out pots, pans, and food storage containers. We eventually had to put locks on the bathroom door and some of the kitchen cabinets.

Shortly after Earnest died, we also learned we had to keep all the outside doors locked. One evening my goddaughter Shawn came to visit us, and while we were in the living room talking, Nate left the room. I thought he had gone to his room. When she left we could not find him anywhere in the house. Stefani and I panicked. I ran outside to look for him, and as I got to the end of the driveway, a man was walking up the street asking if anybody had lost a little boy. I screamed, "Yes!" He told me Nate was down the street at their house. I hollered for Stefani to bring the car and I ran down the street to get him.

We discovered that when Nate left us in the living room, he had opened the side door (which I failed to lock after Shawn came in), and in his pajamas and bare feet, walked down the steps and driveway, made a left turn, walked down our street, and crossed the street to the house which faces perpendicular to our street. This experience taught us we have to make sure all the outside doors are locked while we are in the house, or we will have a run-away child.

Nathan has also kept us very busy and alert because he has quick hands and feet. We cannot leave our food unattended because he may swipe it off our plates and run. Nathan can also challenge us with his stubbornness. For example, when he decides he does not want to get out of the car, he will close the door, and if we reopen the door and unbuckle his seatbelt, he will move to the other side of the car. Some days when he gets off the bus and he does not want to come in the house, he will sit down on the driveway and refuse to move, even when it is cold. The older he gets the stronger and more strong-willed he becomes. We have learned to be creative in our discipline, including time outs and walking away from him. Since he is so loving and sociable, he does not like either form of discipline and will generally cooperate.

Another challenge we faced with Nathan was trying to keep him from pulling at his ears. Since his communication skills were limited, we did not know if he were hurting. He would pull so hard at the back of his ears that he would scratch them raw. This behavior continued through middle school, and affected his ability to wear his hearing aids. Since Nathan's last hearing evaluation in 2007 showed no significant difference in his response to sounds with or without the hearing aids, Nathan no longer wears his hearing aids on a consistent basis.

As Nathan has learned to use his hands more productively, the self stimulating behavior of pulling at his ears has decreased. Rarely does he pull at his ears today; only when he wants immediate attention does he reach for his ears.

Although Nathan's expressive language is still limited, his receptive language is excellent. He can follow simple commands like, "bring me the phone", "take this to your room", "pick this up", and "turn the light on", etc. He also picks up the phone when it rings and knows when doors are opened and closed in the house. Nathan's initial diagnosis of being profoundly deaf has changed to a mild to moderate hearing loss for sound awareness, according to his latest hearing evaluation. Nobody but God could perform that miracle since the nerves in Nathan's inner ear never fully developed.

Nathan can also say specific words such as, "bye-bye", "come on", "momma", "my momma", "papa", "bro-bro", and "no". He has even amazed us at times with two-to-three word sentences such as, "Where's my momma?", "Wasn't me", or "Go Bye-Bye." His sign language vocabulary is also increasing.

For a child whose initial diagnosis was not very promising, Nathan has made amazing progress. He responds to routine and order. Before he leaves home, the lights and TV must be turned off. Before he eats, he must wash his hands and have a napkin at his seat. Cabinet doors must be shut and everything put in place. He pays close attention to where everything is kept and will help put things back in place. He likes to help make the bed, put the laundry in the dryer, empty the trash and replace trash bags in the garbage cans. When he wants to see something different on the TV, he will give us the remote control to change the station or push the buttons himself until the program he wants appears. The news, Wheel of Fortune, and Jeopardy are some of his favorite programs. He also enjoys watching football games and other action sports.

Nathan is now 14, weighs 86 pounds and is 4'8" tall. He is strong as a bull, quite strong-willed and often challenges our patience. There are times when Nate is determined to have things his way whether he is at home, school, church or wherever he goes, earning him the nicknames of "the great manipulator" or "Buster". Although his expressive language is limited, he knows how to get what he wants.

Undoubtedly, Nathan is smart. Once he learns a routine, he remembers it and often resists changing it. He is very observant. For example, he knows when he is going specific places and recognizes destinations. "Go bye -bye" is his favorite phrase and he enjoys riding in any vehicle. Sometimes, he does not want to get off the school bus or out of the car. Whenever Edwin comes to the house, Nate thinks it is time for him to go "bye-bye"; he will grab his hat and his shoes. We have to remind him that every time his brother comes home, it does not mean he is going bye-bye. Nathan also enjoys shopping in the grocery store, pushing the cart, and will fill it if he is not watched. On the other hand, he will also take items out we put in.

In his short life span Nathan has overcome many challenges. He truly is a miracle child whom God chose to demonstrate his power and promises. One of the promises God gave me when I was pregnant was Isaiah 44:24-25:

"I am the Lord who has made all things, who alone stretched out the heavens, who spread out the earth by myself, who foils the signs of false prophets and makes fools of diviners, who over-throws the learning of the wise and turns it into nonsense."

Nathan has baffled many in the medical profession because God has "overthrown the learning of the wise and turned it into nonsense." Things Nathan was not expected or predicted to do, he can do. Nathan can walk, run, climb stairs independently, and do somersaults. He can hear and respond to simple commands. After four years of g-tube feedings, Nathan can eat regular food and drink liquids from a cup without worry of aspiration. He loves to eat, and his appetite is so great that his Granny says she would rather clothe him than feed him. She often wonders if he has two stomachs.

Nathan Lee Benefield is truly a miracle child, who is walking, and communicating via sign language and limited verbal skills. He is healthy and progressing. Only God could touch him and allow him to develop as he has. Through love, prayer and family commitment, Nathan has received the best services and participates in various activities. He has traveled across the state of Georgia and to several other states via car and plane, visiting Disney World, Sea World, Busch Gardens, Hilton Head Island, Myrtle Beach, and the Georgia and Tennessee Aquariums. For two years he has participated in the "Miracle League" at Welcome All Park where children and young adults with special needs learn to play softball. He also enjoys playing basketball.

We praise God for sending Nathan to our family. We love him dearly; he has taught us unconditional love and that love conquers all. Many of us have learned to love in spite of what things appear to be and in spite of the circumstances. The chords of love have bound us closer together.

Not only does our family love him, but our church family has embraced and loved Nathan, even when he turns the lights off in the buildings and runs. They have loved, encouraged, and prayed for us and with us through all of his challenges.

Nathan has been a catalyst to strengthen my faith walk and that of many others. It would have been so easy to worry during my pregnancy and afterwards, but I have learned to trust God. One specific scripture the Lord gave me to diminish worry and fear was Philippians 4:6-7:

"Do not be anxious about anything, but in everything, by prayer and petition, with thanksgiving, present your requests to God. And the peace of God which transcends all understanding will guard your hearts and minds in Christ Jesus."

By internalizing this scripture and Isaiah 44: 24-25, I have found an indescribable peace. Even as we made major decisions regarding his medical care, surgeries, and school placement, I continually believed and held fast to these scriptures.

During these past 14 years, I have seen the power of love and prayer demonstrated over and over again. Because of Nathan, many people have embraced our family with love and prayer; hundreds of people across these United States have prayed for him. The miracles God has performed in his life have strengthened the faith of believers and caused unbelievers to think twice about a God who "can".

We do not know what the future holds for Nate, but we do know who holds his future. Our commitment is to provide the most loving and nurturing environment for Nathan, our gift from God. We have learned unconditional love and how to celebrate even the small miracles of life. The challenges of this journey have been shared by many who desired for Nathan to have a quality life, and we are exceptionally grateful to everyone who worked toward that goal.

This book is the beginning of ***Nathan's Story***. Although Nathan has progressed through the years, I do not know if he will ever be able to live independently because his skills are still limited. So the journey continues with a strong faith in God, love in our hearts and a life-long commitment to care for our very special miracle child.

LESSONS LEARNED FROM NATE & SPECIAL MOMENTS

—⚏—

"My frame was not hidden from you when I was made in the secret place. When I was woven together in the depths of the earth, your eyes saw my unformed body. All the days ordained for me were written in your book before one of them came to be." **(Psalm 139:15-16)**

The two biggest lessons I learned from Nate are about God. When I was younger, I used to always ask for a little brother. So I learned God always answers prayer. It may not be exactly like you want it, but He will still give you what you ask for.

Secondly, I learned that God is really real because after Nate was born some doctors predicted he would not talk or walk. Through the years, even though it has taken some time, Nate hears, he understands, he verbalizes a few words, and he walks. So when the medical people give a diagnosis, they are not always correct. Through prayer anything is possible.

Nate has also helped me with my patience. I have been an impatient person, but in dealing with Nathan I have learned to be patient.

Edwin L. Benefield, Brother

Nathan is a very good communicator and we can all learn from him. Although his verbal skills are limited, he knows how to get his point across. For instance, when I am bouncing a ball, if he wants me to keep bouncing, he will pat his hands on his knees for me to do it again.

Nate is also very observant and very clever. A few times he's had some things in his hands he shouldn't. When I told him to put it down he would drop it to his side on the floor, and then look at me as if to say, "I don't have anything in my hands." One time we actually heard him say, "Wasn't me." I have learned that my little brother Nathan, with his disability, is actually much smarter than the medical profession expected and he continues to baffle some people.

Stefani L. Benefield, Sister

Nate is very loving and he likes to be hugged. He is very attached to me and my wife calls him my shadow because he likes to follow me everywhere I go. Although Nate cannot talk, he observes a lot. Once he learns a routine he doesn't forget it, like the bath process and the routine for getting his breakfast. He can take orders and follow them; he understands directions. Nathan is smart and he knows how to communicate even though his speech is limited.

Rev. Rudolph Smith, Papa

Nate is smart and knows how to avoid discipline. One day when he was smaller and got into trouble, he ran into the bedroom, climbed on the bed and sat among the dolls like he was a doll. I guess he thought I would not recognize him. Now when he does something wrong and knows he will get into trouble, Nate will run into the bathroom, pull his pants down and sit on the commode. That's his tactic to escape punishment since most times he does not use the bathroom independently.

Nathan is his Papa's shadow. One Sunday when my husband was the guest preacher at a church, Nate followed him to the pulpit and sat down beside him until he finished preaching. When the DVD was given to us from the service and we tried to get Nate to watch it, he refused. He knew that he was wrong and did not want to watch it. He knows when he has done wrong. I have learned that even though Nathan has a disability, he knows right from wrong.

Edna L. Smith, Granny

You cannot make Nate do anything that he does not want to and he learns best from repetition. He responds better to you when you speak softly to him and he ignores you when you holler at him. Nate associates certain things with certain people. When you do not respond to what he wants to do, he will give you the bathroom sign because he knows you will get up. I have learned Nate has a mind of his own and knows how to get what he wants, when he wants it.

Auntie Willie Maude Smith – great aunt

Before Nate could walk he learned to climb up on my coffee table. He has shown us how to really love because he is so loving. He always gives me a hug and a kiss.

Louise Knowles (Big Mama) – Great grandmother

Size ain't everything. Nate is strong as a bull. He is a charmer – Smith womanizer – smart and knows how to get what he wants. I have learned strength has nothing to do with size.

Uncle "B" – Leon B. Smith, Jr.

I have had the pleasure of being in Nathan's company on several occasions. What a joy to be in his presence; he has such an enthusiastic spirit and radiates his unconditional love to all around him. As I watch Nathan's family surround him, providing him with the assistance to do things he is unable to do for himself and encouraging him to attempt the tasks they know he can accomplish, it is obvious where his joy, spirit and unconditional love originate.

What is truly remarkable about Nathan is his "Mother"! She is truly the "special" person in Nathan's life. God, in His infinite wisdom, knew she would be the one person in the entire world with patience, understanding, and tireless dedication to fulfill Nathan's needs. For her to be entrusted with the job of raising Nathan is a position of great distinction and honor. As the mother of a special child myself, I know that I too was chosen for all the attributes mentioned above. While I am sure that many challenges and triumphs will be told as *"Nathan's Story"* evolves, let us not forget that there would be no *"Story"* if not for Cheryl and Earnest.

Ramona Burnett (cousin)
Maryland

Nathan,

I first heard about you when you were yet in your mother's womb. She shared with me that you were not well. After you were born, I first saw you in your mother's arms in her bedroom. You were so still and made not a sound. I was surprised to say the least…maybe shocked. Many thoughts ran through my mind, but the one thought that lingered was, this is God's doing, this is God's child, and it's all good.

Nate, you have helped me to be more prayerful and trusting of God. Thank you! As I have watched you these 14 years, I say as the Psalmist, "Great is God and greatly to be praised".

Nathan Benefield, a gift to the Benefield Family, the Smith Family and the Community Church of God Family, as you continue to grow and develop according to God's will, it is my prayer that these families grow and develop along with you according to God's will.

I love you,
Auntie Irma Sanders– great-great aunt

What I learned from Nathan is that love at first sight can last…

Nathan Lee Benefield and I had an encounter of the spiritual kind at Community Church of God back in 1994. It started at the very moment his mom let me hold the little boy bundled up in the blanket. At the time, there was more blanket than baby boy. He was fragile and wobbly, but oh so addictive.

On the very last pew of the church, there we sat. Neither one of us had a care in the world at that moment. Church was over and everyone around us was darting here and there to catch up with this one and that one before they got away. Not us. He was looking up at me and I was looking down at him and we were both trying to figure out who we were and what was going on. Whatever it was, it was happening to both of us because from the outset, Nathan and I connected. I had no clue what to do and he had no clue what I was going to do but nonetheless, we began to do what needed to be done.

Anyone who was involved with the Smith-Benefield clan in those early years will recall how the first few years were touch and go, hope and pray, watch and believe, and see what we would see since none of us knew what the next step would be. There were surgeries and hospital stays, trips to see doctors and specialists, questions about how do you use this machine and when does he get this medicine, and "Is today speech, physical or occupational therapy?"

But let's go back to the beginning, shall we? We began our special journey as godmother and godson when he was dedicated to God on the second Sunday of October in 1994. Like Sarai in the Old Testament who had a child in her old age and became Sarah, I went from Peaches to Godmama because I too had a child of promise in my life (stop worrying about how aged I was).

I was determined that even though we were being told one thing and then another about this limitation and that inability, we were going to do just what pleased us and would be best for him. When he was just a little fella, he and I began to have our one-on-one experiences that made many just shake their heads in disbelief. He and I went there…all by ourselves. I was devoted and dedicated to exposing him to everything the world had to offer, despite what the predictions were. Despite what the doctors said, despite the fact that he couldn't hear nor speak, I was doing it all just because of who he was in my life…my godson.

Even as this chapter of his life is written, we are continuously astounded by Nathan and his ability to be cute as a button, slippery as a snake, and sly as a fox. Like the professionals, sometimes we're confounded and sometimes we realize that he just out manipulates us.

Peaches Moss, Godmother

When Cheryl was pregnant with Nate and learned he had Down syndrome, I thought, "Lord, please give Cheryl and her family the strength they will need." Then Nate was born and Cheryl brought him to Avondale High School. Not only was he a blessing, a gift, and so precious, here was this little person who needed so much love and attention, and he was given to the right family. As we know *God makes no mistakes*!

Jeri Crumley
Former co-worker of Cheryl's

The main thing Nathan taught me was **"patience"** because I remember him as a strong willed child, but also very loving with the support and encouragement from his entire family.

My most outstanding memory of Nathan was when his dad brought him back to see me several years after he graduated from my classroom and moved to another school. (I taught Nathan when he was three to five years of age.) I didn't know they were coming so it was a total surprise when my classroom door opened and Nathan came running in to greet me, but not with words. He circled the room over and over, checking things out thoroughly. He and his dad stayed and visited awhile and when they left, Nathan waved good-bye to me and then proceeded to tell me "bye!"

This amazing memory I will forever cherish because while Nathan was a student in my classroom he neither walked nor talked. So you can understand why there were tears in my eyes as Nathan and his Dad got in their red truck to leave.

Cathy Duncan, Pre- K Teacher

During a week's vacation with Nathan at Hilton Head, I found him to be loving, caring, and quite humorous. I learned to never underestimate his intelligence; for if there were Oscars given for manipulation, Nathan would certainly receive one. He is a master at getting his way unbeknownst to whomever he is dealing with. As long as we were watching him, he would do as he was told. The minute that we would turn our backs he would do what he wanted, whether staying in the pool longer than he was supposed to or not eating his meals. The lesson I learned is that Nathan's disabilities have not hindered him from being in charge of his situations and his surroundings. He is a master at getting his way. I love him.

Rev. L. Pearl Shields
Cleveland, OH

My story is about the time Cheryl invited Shon and me to dinner at her house. When I put my plate down to get something to drink, I did not know how quick Nate was with his hands. He snatched my cornbread, the last piece, and ran. I chased him and then he put the whole piece in his mouth and laughed. All I could say was, "Nate I'm going to get you."

Nate has brought me much happiness when I am around him. He lies down when I blow on his neck and when I stop, he puts his head up again for me to repeat it. Nate, I love you and your family. You have a terrific family and a very special mother who is my special sister and friend.

Minister Maggie Richardson

The lesson I have learned from Nate is how he shows me real love by the way he always hugs and holds onto me. I also admire his sense of "waste" when he turns all the lights off at church.

Maxine Harris

I have learned so much from Nate. Here are some of the lessons I have learned:

- Love is truly unconditional.
- Communication is the backbone of every relationship. Yet, we all don't have to communicate the same way.
- In spite of Nathan's challenges, he is able to break down barriers the speaking population can't.
- You can share your disappointment and continue to have a meaningful relationship with the person who disappointed you.
- Loss is inevitable, but you can grieve and move on with your life. You don't have to become stagnant.
- You can be happy alone when you exercise your mind.
- Set your mind to do what you want to and go after it!

Auntie Sybil O'Neal

Nathan is a testimony that God has created all kinds of people to love. When you get to know Nathan you learn to love him because he loves you in return. Nathan is unique not because of the challenges that make him different, but because of his unique personality. All of us are different and unique.

Nathan likes to have fun. I like to see him laugh. Laughter is an expression that one is having fun. He may not be able to communicate verbally but his communication through laughter lights up a room. Playing with Nathan is a joy especially when he begins to laugh. Laughter is a part of his personality that only those who choose to play with him can experience.

The greatest challenge for family and friends of Nathan is in the area of discipline. None of us likes to constantly discipline him, and sometimes it hurts to do so but he has not yet developed his boundaries. It is my hope that the day will come when we will not have to place him in a chair so that we can control his boundaries. His developing mind has helped him to follow instructions in some areas while we wait for him to mature in other areas.

God loves all of us unconditionally and Nathan is teaching us to love unconditionally. Nathan teaches us patience as we learn to wait on him and serve him. We learn from him servanthood. We also realize that God has a purpose for each of our lives, in spite of our challenges, as he has purpose for Nathan. Nathan has taught us it is important to demonstrate love to one another. He also has taught us persistence because Nathan pursues what he wants. We are grateful that God trusted our family to love one of his special children.

Pastor Michael A. Smith, Uncle

"Because of the Lord's great love, we are not consumed, for His compassions never fail. They are new every morning; great is your faithfulness." (**Lamentations 3:22-23**)

Nathan Lee Benefield, my gift from God, has fulfilled the prophecy spoken over him even when he was in my womb. Two persons prophesied that he would be a strong warrior for the Lord. After he was born, before I knew he was diagnosed as profoundly deaf, God gave me a little melody to sing to him while he was in NICU. It simply said, *"Nathan Lee, Gift of God; Prophecy, Strong Warrior in the Lord."*

During these past 14 years I have learned that Nathan is a strong warrior. His verbal skills may be limited but he knows how to get my attention when he wants something. When he is determined to have his way, Nate can also be a "con artist". In the past few years he has become more strong-willed and stronger, and I have learned different discipline strategies and to pray for wisdom in disciplining him.

Nathan has taught me patience and how to wait on God's timing. His developmental delays provided opportunities for God to place people in my life who encouraged and told me they believed Nathan would eventually walk and talk. It took six and a half years, but he learned to walk. And for a child who was initially diagnosed as profoundly deaf, his receptive language is amazing.

I now know Nathan is an answer to prayer. Early in 1994, my family was going through a crisis and I prayed and asked God for divine intervention. Six weeks later, at age 41, I found out I was pregnant. When the nurse broke the news to me, I cried because I already had two children, ages 16 and 11, and my song had been "two and thru." Later, after Nathan was born, God reminded me that Nathan had not come for me, but for the family. He was the answer to my prayer and truly Nathan has brought our family closer together. His loving disposition makes him so easy to love, and he is the role model for us to love each other unconditionally.

Every night before Nate goes to sleep I anoint him with oil and pray over him. Some mornings he sits on his bed and babbles. It seems as if he is praying, and usually he will not move or come out of his room until he has finished. I believe Nate has a special relationship with God, and I have learned to allow him this time to express himself.

Perhaps one of the greatest lessons I have learned is to allow the tears to flow when I feel overwhelmed, and to surround myself with people who love, encourage, support and pray for me. I have learned to let my mask down, and that it is okay to share my feelings of despondency and fears of the unknown with those who love me. To be emotionally healthy, I needed to let them "in".

Finally, I have learned the power of exceptional parent advocacy. Although, I had always been an advocate for my two older children, I learned I had to advocate more for Nathan. So, I want to encourage all parents to be an exceptional advocate for their special needs child because parent advocacy is vital and essential to procure the necessary services and resources for these children. No one else will fight for your child like you can, so get involved. Ask questions, keep good records and files, contact organizations, seek resources and referrals, and make yourself available to others who may have children with the same or similar diagnosis as yours.

My son, Nathan, the little angel whom God sent us, has shown all who meet him and know him that ***"with God all things are possible."*** His life has touched many people who have learned various lessons from him. For some their faith and prayer life has increased; for others they have learned the meaning of unconditional love. Without a doubt, Nathan is a miracle child who has taught us many lessons.

Cheryl Louise Smith Benefield, Mother

EPILOGUE

—⁓—

"Trust in the Lord with all your heart and lean not on your own understanding; in all your ways acknowledge Him and He will make your paths straight." **(Proverbs 3:5-6)**

My hope is that after reading **Nathan's Story** you will recognize that our journey is God-ordained and that God will perform His word if we believe and trust in Him. As in all journeys, our family encountered some curves, potholes and detours, but God always brought us through. Nathan's life is a testimony that God is real and He still performs miracles.

Truly, Nathan is a blessing to our family, and he has brought us closer to God and to each other. Even in the midst of all the challenges, we have seen God's mighty hand at work. Our greatest challenge now is in the area of discipline. Nathan is very strong, strong willed and determined to have his way. My ninety-five year old Big Mama aptly sums it up when she says, "Sometimes he's so sweet I could eat him up and sometimes he's so bad, I wish I had."

Through all the challenges, I know my faith in God, the love, support and prayers of family and friends have sustained me. During the past twenty plus years two extraordinary women, Bernadine Joubert and Vivian Hall, modeled unconditional love, the power of prayer and exceptional parent advocacy as they raised their special needs sons. I have watched them persevere and overcome challenges, and I am very grateful for their encouragement along my journey.

Finally, I hope **Nathan's Story** encourages you to believe in the almighty God who is *"willing to do and can do"* the miraculous. I pray that as you continue your life's journey that you will know the abiding love of God, the transforming power of prayer, and develop an enduring faith in God which will sustain you through all of life's challenges. May you learn to stand on the promises of God because His word is true. May you be inspired to love all children unconditionally because God loves us unconditionally. Remember, God is faithful and His love never fails. Shalom!

OUR MIRACLE BABY

Before he was born
He was adored.
Even though it was not planned,
I was willing to understand
That with each passing day
Our miracle baby was on the way.

Days turned into weeks,
And weeks into months.
It didn't take long
Before we had a handsome, baby boy.

He was born nine weeks early
Before we expected,
Weighing in at three pounds, 13 ounces
Not much bigger than an ant.

Named Nathan Lee,
My little brother indeed –
I can remember it like it was yesterday
But now he's three.

His name means "*Gift of God*",
And he truly is
Our miracle baby –
Whom we love with all our hearts.

Stefani Benefield
02/1998

Please visit our website at <u>www.ourmiraclechild.</u>
<u>com</u> for additional information.